I0840204

The Keto Diet

Zero to Keto in 30 Days

By

James King

Copyright © 2019 James King

All rights reserved.

ISBN: 9781698485201

CONTENTS

FOREWARD

The Keto Diet, also known as the Ketogenic Diet, encourages the body to an extreme change in the origin of the primary source of energy.

Many people reach a stage late in their lives where they desire a radical change in their appearance, often defined primarily by the desire to lose weight. Most in this position seek out a diet plan, where you are forced to sacrifice daily by eating next to nothing. At this difficult stage, the truth is that many diets will not guarantee you satisfactory results.

The Keto diet invites you to do what other diets forbid you in excess, it allows the consumption of foods high in fat, and like a sacrifice, all diets have one, it entirely regulates the intake of foods high in carbohydrates.

Of course, you have to be very careful and constant in this diet. Otherwise, it may not work.

In this book, you can find all the information you need to start a Keto diet today, and we will discuss topics such as:

- The correct way to start the Keto diet.
- Foods you can consume.
- Foods you should avoid.
- How to introduce Keto in a non-invasive way.
- And more

vii

CHAPTER 1 – INTRODUCTION TO KETO

The most popular diets often include a high carbohydrate intake and protein moderation combined with partial or total fat removal. This high carbohydrate intake translates into increased glucose, or sugar which is the energy source that the body uses most often.

This occurs because glucose is far easier to produce from carbohydrates. The body will identify carbohydrates already converted to glucose to be of greater importance than consumed fats. By default, this will then cause glucose to be burned as an energy source, and fats to stagnate and remain within the body, which logically will lead to increased weight gain.

Carbohydrates accumulate in the body because when they enter the system and are processed, they are transformed into sugars. These sugars, in turn, provide energy to the body. However, surplus sugars are not discarded. The body seeks to maintain its reserves and changes the remaining sugars into localized fat.

To avoid this, there is a type of diet that promotes the opposite effect. This is the Keto Diet.

What is it?

The ketogenic diet has its origins in the treatment of epileptic patients and derives its name from Dr Russell M. Wilder, a distinguished clinician and scientist. His treatments were mainly based on placing the body in a state of ketosis, the state that derives from the lack of energy reserves previously mentioned.

Ketosis can manifest itself through fasting, although if you want good results this method is not recommended. Another way in which a state of ketosis can be reached is through organizing food consumption. To do this, you must regulate a frequent energy source such as carbohydrates, whilst adding another less common source, such as fat.

The Keto diet, as mentioned before, consists of high fat intake, eliminating carbohydrates and moderating proteins. This diet also benefits people who have flour allergies, since eliminating carbohydrates is gluten-free. Pasta, bread, cakes, rice, potatoes and all carbohydrates are eliminated from the diet; which in turn causes the body to eliminate all the remaining stored glucose.

By running out of carbohydrates, the system will begin a search for energy. Since only fat is consumed, it will be interpreted that this is now your primary source of energy. The priority given to that causes stored fat to become consumed from now on, provoking the state known as ketosis.

During ketosis the fat will begin to break down into ketones, supplying the energy required by the system. Put simply, ketosis will help you burn all the stored fat that had accumulated over long periods adopting incorrect diets and ill-advised lifestyle choices.

As your body eliminates fat during ketosis, you will lose weight quicker than using any other diet. It will also provide many benefits, such as no excessive hunger during the diet; leading to a more satisfying state of well being. An additional benefit is you will lose weight without the need for hard exercise or incorporating calisthenics into your daily routines to achieve your goals.

While it is true that exercise is quite beneficial for weight loss, the ketogenic diet will help you avoid the necessity for it.

This type of diet should be carried out following plans established by a nutritionist. Otherwise, it could have repercussions if done without guidance. So if you are considering applying it, you must follow specific guidelines that you can understand and pursue over the course of the diet.

CHAPTER 2 – KETO DIET MENU COMPOSITION

The ketogenic diet menu is based upon high fat and no carbohydrates. Those who wish to apply should follow a list of foods that have been verified by a nutritionist so that this type of diet does not adversely affect their metabolism or health.

Under a ketogenic diet, you cannot consume all types of fat, as there are some fats that regardless of diet will prove harmful. It is important to follow a specific menu so as not to make mistakes such as confusing these fats.

Additionally, carbohydrates and any food rich in sugars should be completely eliminated from consumption, so that fats and proteins take prominence within the daily menu.

A solely Keto diet can be adopted for a period of 1 month to a maximum of 3 months. Following this period, a carbohydrate diet should be resumed so as to not excessively or permanently disrupt the body's metabolism. However, as an alternative option, the keto diet can be performed intermittently.

This intermittent form is called a cyclic ketogenic diet, which consists of for every five days of a consecutive diet, two carbohydrate meals are included. This modality does not have a maximum established duration since in this way carbohydrate intake is regulated within the diet to not produce damage to the metabolism.

Here are some ideas for your daily meals, including not only breakfast, lunch and dinner but also some snacks between these meals:

Breakfast
Undoubtedly the most important meal of the day, breakfast must be given a special priority. It is important not to be hungry during the morning, while conversely, not to consume more than you should.

To start your day with the most energy, we recommend two fried eggs with two slices of bacon, accompanied by a cup of tea or coffee without sugar. Remember, as sugars are a source of glucose, concentrated sources should not be consumed. In addition to this, you can complement your morning dish with half a cup of blueberries or raspberries.

If this seems somewhat repetitive, another option is to make a sandwich... without bread. To clarify, it is suggested that you substitute the bread with fried eggs, using them as the top and bottom of the sandwich, which can then be stuffed with ham, salami, cheese, or avocado.

Although this type of breakfast can be quite significant to your daily routine, it should be complemented with a snack mid-morning. We suggest a handful of nuts of your choice; such as almonds or peanuts. Another option you can safely add is yoghurt, so long as it is of a natural flavour without added sugar.

Lunch

While breakfast may undoubtedly be the most important meal of the day, lunch should always be the most substantial. So while despite the fact we are on a diet, this should be one of the daily meals that are best tailored to suit us. To have lunch like a king and not be hungry at any time in the afternoon, here are some dishes for you to enjoy or be inspired by.

For a pleasant way to enjoy lunch on the Keto diet, you can try grilled salmon bathed in mustard. As an accompaniment to this excellent mid-day meal, you can partake in an arugula and cucumber salad, with a dressing of mayonnaise, garlic and extra virgin olive oil.

For a follow-up snack, a good idea is a cup of 8 strawberries or raspberries slices alongside some natural yoghurt and sesame seeds.

Dinner

Generally, dinner is characterized by being the heaviest meal of the day, however, in this case, it will be equally as bulky as lunch. This is because while you sleep the body goes into a more in-depth process of nutrient breakdown. Because of this, the last two dishes must be of considerably larger amounts, in addition to being higher in fat so that ketosis is quickly established.

For a Keto dinner, you can include two beef fillets, with a four-cheese sauce consisting of Mozzarella, Gruyere, Roquefort and Parmesan. This dish can be elegantly served on a bed of Asparagus and Paprika Julienne sautéed with Butter.

It is recommended that following dinner, a period of rest is taken, a little before going to bed, to make certain the body is in a more calm state to sleep. This is done so that the body properly breaks down food without interference.

CHAPTER 3 – FOOD ALLOWED

To perform the Keto diet, it is important to know the foods that you can eat so that no random elements are introduced during it. Foremost any foods containing glucose must be eliminated, specifically, sugar derivatives. Likewise, you should ignore the consumption of carbohydrates entirely.

Red meat

The Keto diet does not prohibit proteins in their entirety, and one source you can safely eat that does not interfere with ketosis is red meat.

Red meats that you can consume must be organic or grass-fed meats, as these are the healthiest. They can be eaten baked, roasted, grilled and even in salads.

Fish

Another food allowed for ketosis to properly occur is fish. Fish can be eaten, boiled, grilled, fried, smoked or baked. The main recommended fish is salmon as it is high in fat, however, you can also opt for cod, tuna or even mackerel.

Vegetables

Although it may not seem like it, there are many vegetables that cannot enter the Keto diet under any circumstances. This is because despite being health-promoting, there are still some vegetables quite high in carbohydrates; such as potatoes.

Within the Keto diet, the only allowed vegetables for consumption are grown on the surface, not underground. Vegetables that are available for the ketogenic diet are Cauliflower, Brussel Sprouts, Spinach, Broccoli, Cabbage and even Avocado.

These do not necessarily have to be boiled or made in salads, and you can also choose to cook them sautéed in butter or in the oven with abundant extra virgin olive oil.

Eggs

Eggs are another high source of protein equally as important as meat or fish. These have great versatility in the kitchen; being a food allowed in the diet helps to not have significant limitations while preparing replacement recipes.

Eggs can be fried, boiled, poached, scrambled, beaten, prepared in omelettes, in butter and even in soup.

Dairy products

Generally, these products are high in fat; this is a point in their favour within the Keto diet. It will be necessary to consume as much fat as possible so that the diet works correctly to establish ketosis as soon as possible.

The dairy products that are allowed to be ingested are butter, cheese, and even high-fat yoghurts lacking added sugars. Sour cream also has its place on the Keto menu. Milk must be consumed very moderately, as it contains carbohydrates; and only whole milk should be ingested.

Nuts

Nuts, peanuts, hazelnuts, pine nuts, almonds and Brazil nuts are the most recommended nuts to consume on a Keto diet. Even though they are allowed, they should be ingested with caution, since some can be transformed into glucose if their consumption in excessive amounts.

Butters derived from these nuts can also be implemented within the diet. However, these should be high in fat, without carbohydrates or added sugars.

Fruits

Most fruits are high in carbohydrates, due to their sugar and glucose levels. Citrus fruits or berries are the best options to include in a Keto diet.

Recommended fruits, as they are low in carbohydrates, are plums, blueberries, raspberries, blackberries, strawberries, blackberries, cherries and even peaches in a few portions. You can also cook with lime or lemon if you wish since they do not contain many carbohydrates, and if you like coconut, you can eat their meat as a snack.

Natural fats

The main factors in the ketogenic diet are fats, and the highest nutrient intake of the diet should be from fats. However, not all fats are suitable for a Keto diet.

The fats you can safely consume are butter, olive oil, coconut oil, mayonnaise, cream cheese, sour cream, spicy tabasco sauce, soy sauce and even guacamole.

Drinks

Most soft drinks are rich in carbohydrates, not to mention high in sugars. Due to this your most reliable option should always be water, with ice or without ice. If this seems too simple for your palette, you can add lemon drops or slices of lime.

On the other hand, if you're a fan of hot drinks, specifically coffee, don't worry. Coffee does not have carbohydrates, so you can have pleasant breakfasts under the condition you do not use sugar in it. It is worth noting milk should not be added either due to its carbohydrates. Alternatives are black tea, green tea, white tea and chamomile.

Finally, there is tea, and just like coffee it should be kept glucose-free, and without sugars. On the other hand, you can add lemon or lime drops to make it more palatable.

CHAPTER 4 – FORBIDDEN FOOD

As is well known, the Keto diet strictly prohibits the consumption of carbohydrates. Mainly because they interfere with the ketosis process and prevent it from happening. However, common carbohydrates are not the only foods you should avoid when adopting the ketogenic diet.

Fat

Although the Keto diet is mainly composed of fats, there are very high carbohydrate fatty products. These logically must be avoided at all costs. To prevent mistakes, you must be clear about these types of fat.

With vegetable oils, you should avoid consuming soy, canola, corn, grapeseed, sunflower, sesame and peanut oils.

Also, you should eliminate the consumption of processed foods, such as sausages, fast food, ice cream, wheat gluten, cookies, chocolate, margarine, cakes, doughnuts, cereals, sports drinks, sodas, beers, fruit juices and sweets.

Dairy products

Although some cheeses and small portions of natural yoghurt enter the diet, there are some dairy products that should be left off the menu. This can be caused by two factors, by their carbohydrates or by their sugars.

First, you should avoid any milk that is not complete, that is, skimmed, semi-skimmed, chocolate, with artificial flavours and all those that do not meet that characteristic and are carbohydrate-rich.

In addition to this, the only yoghurt that can be consumed is natural yoghurt or Greek yoghurt. It is also advised that you should avoid eating cheese as a snack constantly; this can easily be transformed into glucose.

Cereals

This seemingly harmless group of foods contain the highest percentage of carbohydrates. Mainly for wheat, from which flour is derived, the primary source of carbohydrates such as pasta, bread, cakes and dough in general. This is why cereals containing gluten should be avoided. Rice can be a complement to foods that do not follow a Keto diet, so it also evades. Oatmeal is another cereal that cannot be included in the ketogenic diet along with rye and barley.

Vegetables

Although these are an excellent complement in a daily dish, some are very high in carbohydrates; logically, they should not be included within the Keto diet.

The prohibited legumes are white beans, lentils, chickpeas, black beans and green peas.

Starches

There is a temptation to include starches to help keep you full; either a piece of bread to a bag of crisps. These are the foods that are commonly consumed and convenient, however, should be avoided the most. bread, pasta, potatoes and their derivatives, carrots and cassava.

Sugars

Glucose is the number one enemy of ketosis. Therefore, you should not consume anything that has sugar, or its derivatives, since this will alter the ketogenic process.

It should be noted that sweeteners are not to be used in any form; aspartame, sugaring, sucralose, Splenda and acesulfame should not be consumed for any reason.

Fruits

By their nature, fruits contain glucose; that is, they are sweet. Therefore they should not be included within an effective Keto diet. However, not all fruits are prohibited.

You should avoid mainly bananas, watermelons, grapes, oranges, pineapples, apples and all their juices, especially those that are concentrated.

CHAPTER 5 – KETO BENEFITS

Once your body is in Ketosis you can expect to experience weight loss, fat accumulated over the years will be burned through. However, there are benefits that go beyond removing a couple of kilos to the balance.

In addition to significant health benefits and functionality for disease treatments, the Keto diet also helps your body's image in different aspects.

The multiple advantages of applying a ketogenic diet are divided into two branches. The aesthetic benefits and medicinal benefits.

Aesthetic Benefits

The ketogenic diet not only delivers benefits to your health but are also aesthetic in nature. It should be noted that indirectly these benefits are also beneficial for your health. However, the main ones are the anti-ageing control, the loss of fat and the recovery of healthier skin.

Ageing control

The body accelerates the ageing process by eating a high-calorie diet. With a diet based on carbohydrates, without the restriction of glucose levels and in addition to the excessive consumption of fat in a state in which there is no ketosis the body will be in need of manufacturing and reusing new cells.

This is because you cannot process all carbohydrates and fats with existing cells. Through this cycle, the ageing of the person will begin more quickly. This will result in him not being able to perform many of his vital functions. Therefore, it will start to generate failures.

Thanks to the Keto diet, the body can process more efficiently all the nutrients consumed. Additionally, it will protect from some metabolic disorders and any derivations that are harmful to health.

Fat loss

The accumulation of fats throughout the body has always been one of the biggest concerns of people in terms of aesthetics. The ketogenic diet, as explained above, eliminating carbohydrates will cause the body to directly consume accumulated fat stores. Eliminating with it a percentage of the total body mass of the body. This can be expressed in abdominal fat or even cellulite.

Recovery of skin health

Pimples, pimples and acne are inflammations that are generated from defence against insulin. As the Keto diet is well known to release ketones, ketones have anti-inflammatory abilities. This will benefit all those people who suffer from acne or some type of inflammatory skin condition, allowing it to disappear.

Medicinal benefits

As already mentioned, the Keto diet or at least a similar concept was originated to treat patients with epilepsy. However, the ketogenic diet not only brings benefits to treat epilepsy, but there are also interesting advantages such as improved mood, improved cognitive skills and improved immune system.

Mood improvement

By having a diet high in carbohydrates, the body will always be involved in a kind of constant repetition. This cycle is due to the fact that the consumption of carbohydrates and glucose can be reflected as an addiction. Not only that but if you continue to maintain this type of eating habit it will not satisfy your hunger and often induce cravings.

The addiction to caloric foods can produce anxiety and stress, leading to mood swings that are easily avoidable. Through the ketogenic diet, the metabolism is stabilised, the constant feeling of hunger is eliminated, and finally, your good mood is restored.

Improves cognitive skills

Thanks to the ketones and their constant passage through the blood vessels, it provides the nervous system with a good source of energy. This will significantly improve the enzymatic functions that the brain performs, as well as optimise the work of neurotransmitters.

This will eventually result in your blood vessels having a better flow, allowing you to connect more neurons at the same time. In a way that increases your ability to concentrate and eliminates possible cases of mental fatigue.

It improves the immune system

The Keto diet helps your body get used to burning fat and ketone organisms. Thanks to this, the production of two antioxidant enzymes, Catalase and Glutathione, is increased. These repair from minimal damage generated with day to day to some more severe as oxidative stress.

Thus the ketogenic diet helps not only improve your immune system but also restores and slows the ageing of your cells.

CHAPTER 6 – KETO RECIPES

The ketogenic diet is very beneficial for many aspects. However, it has a degree of complexity, which is the replacement of caloric foods with high-fat ones. In order to properly comply with the Keto diet, we give you two ketogenic recipes for you to enjoy a lunch or dinner and breakfast.

Turkish eggs with yoghurt

This is a recipe to start the day, full of energy and protein, all necessary to be able to perform all morning. Its preparation is very simple. First, beat 120g of Greek yoghurt so that it is creamy, then mixed with herbs of your choice, they can be rosemary, oregano, thyme and coriander.

Then add the black pepper and salt. Subsequently, the yoghurt is placed in a deep bowl leaving a hole in the centre. This will be for poached eggs that are cooked alongside all the previous steps. Finally, the eggs are placed in the centre and a wonderful Keto breakfast is enjoyed.

Microwave Curry Turkey

This idea can be used for a dinner or a Keto lunch. Mainly, it will start by cutting a 500g turkey tenderloin into strips, to season it with salt and pepper, as well as onion in julienne. On the other hand, 250 g of natural yoghurt, 50 g of cream cheese, 50 ml of evaporated milk, two tablespoons of curry powder and chopped coriander to taste will be mixed in a microwave-safe container.

This will be mixed until everything is integrated, then the turkey already seasoned will be added, it will be mixed again well. Once this has been done it will be covered with punctured film paper and cooked in the microwave oven for 800 Watts for 5 minutes. Once you are ready, taste it and enjoy your lunch or dinner, Keto.

CHAPTER 7 – SIMPLE WAYS TO INTRODUCE KETO INTO YOUR LIFE

Having learned what Ketosis is, what ketone organisms are, what the Keto diet entails and what its main characteristics are, you should learn how to start putting it into practice. Even if you have already acquired the know-how and have your weekly menu prepared, entering ketosis is not as easy as it seems.

The Diet becomes difficult if you complicate it by rushing into it blindly without understanding fully, not following the instructions and under-eating. There is a danger of 'Stress Ketosis' this happens because the body detects this stressful situation, protects and preserves all sources of energy that the body has, as it interprets the stress as a safety alert.

This will result in you not burning a gram of fat or going into ketosis. Therefore, you must stay relaxed and stress-free to start dieting.

Some useful tips are; to sleep early and the whole night, enjoy more natural environments to induce relaxation and limit your use of electronic devices and social media.

Once you are stress-free, ensure you set a specific day to start the diet. The previous day you can eat everything that is prohibited in the Keto and abundantly, but only until 5:30 in the afternoon.

This will generate enough energy reserves to support 24 hours of fasting. You will only eat again at dinner time the next day, with a ketogenic menu. That is, you can have coffee or tea during breakfast on the first day. In the case of the second day, you will only skip breakfast. Then on the third day, normal ketogenic status is established.

It should be noted that you can rectify if you are in ketosis by performing a urine test for ketogenic organisms, this will tell you if your work is well done or you should do it again.

CHAPTER 8 – KETO CONTRAINDICATIONS

Although the ketogenic diet can bring a wide variety of benefits, there are some exceptions in which it would not be advisable to attempt the Keto diet. These cases are reflected in those people with high fat intake and those people who depend on a daily carbohydrate diet.

Mainly it should be clear that the diet should not be carried out for more than three continuous months of ketosis. Otherwise, it can drastically disrupt your metabolism.

Those with heart problems should avoid the Keto Diet, as with high-fat consumption, some cases of arrhythmias can occur.

Similarly, pregnant or breastfeeding women should not try this, as, during pregnancy and postpartum, the energy consumption and nutrients required are different.

It should be noted that the ketogenic diet can cause, in any case, cramps, a decline in your physical performance and bad breath. For this reason, we recommend that you analyse all the factors that the diet entails before putting it into practice.

CONCLUSION

The Keto or ketogenic diet enables you to lose weight and accumulated fat, then sustain that loss for several months or even years. The Keto diet is effective because through high fat consumption and eliminating carbohydrates, a state of ketosis is achieved.

This state occurs when the body stops burning its main energy reserves, in this case, carbohydrates and begins to look for another source of food. Since only fat is ingested, the brain will give the order to use the fats to convert to energy. In this way ketones, organisms that supply energy to the body, thus burning the fat accumulated in it are generated.

This will affect a decrease in weight and fat, as well as a decreased appetite and without leaving you feeling hungry. There is no need to count calories or exhaust yourself by over-exercising, just follow the diet.

However, this diet is only recommended for a transitory period of time or failing that, in cycles, which as explained before, consists of consuming ketogenic diet for five days and then two carbohydrates.

If you are considering adopting the Keto Diet, you should always consult with a nutritionist to ascertain if this type of ketogenic diet will be beneficial or if it can harm you. They can advise you which other similar diets to attempt, that offer similar advantages.

www.ingramcontent.com/pod-product-compliance
Lightning Source LLC
Chambersburg PA
CBHW061331250726
48657CB00003B/1112